PRAISE FOR

# 'Tight Buns'

*& fat loss in 30 days or less with flowologee*

"Wow, Sakani!
"Let me start off by saying how happy I am for you.  In my opinion, you are now well on your way to producing a thoughtful and well written plan which will be sure to engage others, motivate others and bring
benefit to others."

"Sakani, I again congratulate you on a wonderful new start."

Kind regards,
Aletia Howard
Owner
So Help Me..."Booktique"
Cleveland, OH

# 'Tight Buns'

*& fat loss in 30 days or less with flowologee*

## Sakani D'Angeles

2013

©

## DBC PUBLISHING GLOBAL

www.sakanidangeles.com

3

Edition: **1**

*Thank you for purchasing my book!*

SUPPORT THE TEACHERS WHO TEACH BENEFICIAL INFORMATION THAT HELP PEOPLE IMPROVE-

5% of all author royalties are donated to educational not-for-profits.

www.sakanidangeles.com

# A story to begin with...

There were 2 doctors measuring the effects of **positive** and **negative** environments on positive and negative children. They took a negative boy and negative girl and placed them in a room of all the best toys. Once the children entered the room they started complaining saying, "this toys is no good, that toy is no good", etc.

They doctors wondered what the positive children were doing because they were placed in a room full of horse *manure*.

The doctors looked into the window of the door and saw the two children wearing yellow rubber boots that reached up to their knees. They had shovels in their hands and they were shoveling the manure around the room enthusiastically with very big smiles on their faces.

The doctors entered the room and asked the children,
"why are you two smiling?"

They said,

"when we saw all this poop... we thought,

## *'there had to be a pony in here somewhere!'*

*This book is your pony and I encourage you to ride it to success!*

# First & Foremost

One day in early 2003 I heard from one of my clients. Regina said that by simply following an earlier version of my step-by-step guide:

*'Tight Buns' & a 'thinner' you in 30 days or less with flowologee*

it made her dream of slimming down and trimming up come true. She went to give me a lot of accolades that made me feel a bit uncomfortable. This happens to me a lot and I wish to be honest with you... the real secret is that *she took action*.

**Taking action** is **99%** of this. This **book** is 1%. Anyone can follow the step-by-step win-win system I have come up with but unfortunately 99% of people are too lazy to do it. So I have created this book and if *you just take action* it should help you prepare for one of the best days of your life!

One question I get a lot is why did I create this book when there are so many other fitness books out there? The answer is pretty easy, but kind of disappointing. Long story short is that I wanted to help people like you who are going through exactly what I went through 8 years ago. I met a lady who I and things proceeded up to where we were planning to get married.

I can't tell you how many women I know have a hard time:

*finding an exercise program that is **easy** to do and that would help them get fit **fast** for the 'Wedding Day'*

*finding an **easy** meal plan to help them fast **without hurting themselves** in the process*

I really *love* to help people and I feel like this is my calling in life. I look forward to hearing your testimonial knowing you found success in getting ready for one of the biggest days of your life... 'the Wedding Day!'

Before we move on let me ask you this, how awesome would it be if there was an exercise program that solved all major problems of weight loss and toning up for the 'Wedding Day?'

- How to think & eat in a way that will have *good* long term effects.
- How to specifically 'enhance' your 'hour glass'.
- How to get a good value *fast* for a fraction of the cost.

Well that would be pretty sweet and I have to tell you since I discovered those items it has been a game changer for me.

The day before I wrote this book I woke up only to be HIT with emails from people who are not even preparing for a wedding and who want my

tips RIGHT NOW!

Ann, a long time friend of mine, *"Sakani, thanks for the 30 day program. People have been asking me what I am doing and my husband has taken notice and has loved the results! So simple, yet so effective-*

*-This is the real deal Sakani!"*

*Brides to be & Brides Maids are going to* **love** *this book!"*

*So I am really excited to finish this book for you 'Bride to be, Brides Maids or you who wish to shape your body & lose weight within 30 days or less!' I am honored with your continued reading of this book! It is vital that you are ready to go.*

# think, be, do, have...?

This book Vol. 1 consists of 2 parts:

## Part 1

### (*think & be*)

Thought comes before action. Most books share with you how to do what needs to be done in order to get the results that you want. The reality is a person is lost if a person doesn't know the proper way to **think** so that they can be consistent and enjoy the results for a long time into the future. The information in this book I have done myself first. My strategy is a good choice for you & it works!

## Part 2

### (*do & have... the program*)

This is where I show the best exercises to shape your body for the 'Day!'

### And...

This is the have section and that is the future and **totally up to you**. If you choose to follow the information in this book that is based on scientific proof and practical application among many people then *you should achieve the results you wish for.* If you decide to alter what is in this book and you get results other than what you are looking for then you are keeping yourself from a *beautiful* goal.... *the goal of enhancing your body.*

# think & be

Most books on eating healthy begin with the *do* and *have* portions of the goal setting method mentioned earlier. The reality is that thinking *always* comes before action. In addition, we should watch the "advice" we take from people and so called experts. Why? Well there are 2 types of people: Mentors-*those who have done what we wish to do* and advisers-*those who tell people what to do and may or may not have done it themselves.* Here is a perfect story that explains the benefits and harms of taking good advice and bad advice.

There was a man who killed 99 people. He felt bad. He went to a man known for how "good" he was. The killer went to the man and told him he felt bad and was there any way to change his ways. The "good" man said, "no." The killer then killed him. The killer still felt bad and kept on searching for the answer to his question.

He came across a "knowledgeable" man and asked him his question sincerely eager in knowing the answer. The "knowledgeable" man told them there was *always* a way out and a way to being better. He told the killer to leave from where he was living and move to a city where everyone was trying to be better. The man left to begin his new life.

There are many benefits to learn from this story. A major benefit is the importance of knowing who to ask for information. A "good" person is different than a "knowledgeable" person. For example a man or woman working out in a gym who looks to be in shape is not necessarily the best person to ask a question about 'your" body and what works for 'you.'

Ask them at your own risk! How many times have we asked someone an exercise or meal question and become unsuccessful after we apply the information they told us? We asked the wrong person. How much time can be saved if we learned a different way to **THINK** about how we approach our health and fitness?

That is a point of difference between myself and other fitness coaches out there in the world. I teach my clients how to *think differently.* This thinking allows them to remain consistent in their efforts. It also allows them to apply or not apply new health and exercise information as they receive it.

Another benefit from the story is knowledge always comes before action. Do you drive from Los Angeles to New York City without looking at map? Why then do we approach healthy eating and fitness with an approach that is similar to throwing food on the wall hoping that some will stick? Have you seen how most people who come to a fitness center to exercise have no paper or pen in their hand? How can they document what they are doing so they can become better?

*"Knowledge before action"* is a motto the most successful people apply and that is where we shall begin in this book and we shall end in this book with a simple explanation of how to eat to increase your energy. I have included simple charts you can print out and place where you can view them whenever you eat.

Another benefit is the understanding that "lack of knowledge is a sickness." In order to better understand what must be done we must look at the symptoms of the "sickness."

What are the *symptoms*?

Buying anything that looks like it will help one lose weight or a new exercise regimen getting no results.

What is the *cause*?

Opportunistic thinking.

What is the healthy weight and exercise **problem**?

Lack of a Strategy.

The reality of our life when it comes to seeking good health is that there *are*

# 2 types of people:

## Opportunity Fitness Seekers
*A new video on how to lose weight appears on late night television and you purchase it.*

Most people who struggle with their weight and healthy eating are busy with the day to day activities of their life and they take action and buy those things that appeal to their emotions.

## Strategic Fitness Thinkers
*You have a vision of how you wish to feel, how you wish to look and what you wish to do... and a fitness and healthy eating goal in mind.*

Successful people who have reached and are setting new healthy eating and fitness goals *know* their vision, develop many paths to reach their goals and choose the approach that is the best. The continually ask "what are the best paths to help me get better physically?"

# Poor strategy results in you losing confidence and then stopping the progress to your goals... again.

# Opportunity Fitness Seekers

An Opportunity Fitness Seeker is *always* looking for the next big "weight loss" video, book or website. The only question they ask is "Can I lose weight with this?" So today it is this diet, tomorrow that diet and so on. They buy many programs, books, vitamins, join many associations and only consistently apply a few of them. They get rid of the old one when the new program comes along.

# Strategic Fitness Thinkers

A Strategic Fitness Thinker operates with a different question in their minds. "Will this new program help me get closer to my goal?" That is what they ask. They have a clear vision of how they want their body to look and how they want to feel. They can analyze their own strengths and study different strategies.

They make an educated decision after studying the new information and then apply the information in a way that helps them progress further and closer to their *"vision"* and *goal*. A Strategic Fitness Thinker knows that their biggest opportunity is inside of themselves: *following their ideal strategy* and not the hot product of the day, week, month or year.

Here is a secret that you are *not* supposed know: It is easier to sell an **Opportunity Fitness Seeker** than it is to sell a Strategic Fitness Thinker. Why? The Opportunity Fitness Seeker has no criteria-if you can convince them that they will lose weight and shape the body of their dreams then you have made your sale! A **Strategic Fitness Thinker** compares what you are offering to their current strategy-*will it help me get better without* losing progress?

**W**ill it help them in some way? Will it help them to get to their body shape faster? Will it help them have more energy? Will it help them to sleep better? Will it help them stay away from the caffeinated drinks and pills that give artificial energy?

Is it information that fits into their current strategy and if it does is it superior to what they are doing now? *Here is the thing... Here it is*. Most people that go to fitness centers are Opportunity Fitness Seekers. They have no strategy, they jump from fad and diet to fad and diet and while they have *some* success with their bodies they have no vision of the overall fitness strategy they would need to create in order to achieve it.

And another thing... here is the thing. Since they do not have a *clear* vision they are not able to follow any sort of detailed plan to accomplish it. As a result they end up buying anything and everything that comes with the *promise* of easy results! They really *love* the "results in a box" products where the promises are large with little to no effort! (Including weight loss 'clothes!')

If you we were to look at the behavior of most people who exercise and try to eat right wouldn't you agree that they have been subconsciously following the strategy of adding more and more methods?

# What's next?

What follows are the "how" part of this book. I have created some easy to apply charts and a VERY SIMPLE set of instructions. This book was designed on purpose to be the size of a normal page of paper so you take it right to a copy machine and make copies of the charts or cut them right out and place them where you can be reminded and guided. No complex eating, counting calorie stuff here...

I wish you to have TIME to do the things you wish and standing around counting calories will *waste your time*... No disrespect to those who do... This is a different approach... Let's begin...

# Now...

There was a doctor named Dr. Arthur Steinhaus (1897–1970). He created this program called "Peripheral Heart Action." It was the predecessor to circuit training. His version explained that a person would stay at a station or exercise for 30 to 60 seconds doing as many reps as he or she could and then without stopping would move to the next exercise in the workout.

**Four things would happen in this workout:**

1.) Their heart rate would be elevated and the blood as a result of moving from exercise to exercise would strengthen the heart itself thereby increasing cardiovascular endurance.

2.) The muscles of the body itself would get stronger as a result of using weights during each exercise.

3.) Flexibility would improve as a result of stretching AFTER and only AFTER the workout.

4.) Fat loss would increase resulting in a more defined look.

I have modified the workout by adding some research of my own based on my own exercises experiences traveling across America while working in logistics with an Import/Export company. Constantly traveling without access to a gym or fitness center caused me to look for ways to maintain and increase my physical ability without wearing me out in the process. I identified exercise bands as the most efficient due to the fact that I could put them in a back pack. My version eliminated the need to do cardio exercise since at its core it is a complete workout. I call it:

# flowologee

"the art of enhancing the human body"

The **best** body part exercise order to **tighten** your buns & **lose fat** is:

## LEGS

## SHOULDERS

## BACK

## BICEPS

## TRICEPS

# Why this order?

Muscle & Fitness magazine published the findings of research in 2007 which order of exercises are good for the body. They found that this order gives the body rest so you are able to go from one body part to the next _without_ the body getting tired. More importantly, your body is able to bring all **100%** of effort to the exercise and that should result in you looking **fantastic** by the end of the 30 days!

The objective is to do the suggested circuits or "flows" in 30 minutes **MAX**.

# There is no need to go past 30 minutes!

One small **Hollywood** proof in addition to the scientific proof that can be verified?

In an interview with **Men's Health**, we learn about Mark Wahlberg:

_"Even now that he's a mega-star, his focus still remains. As for his workout, Mark believes in keeping it simple. For 30 minutes a day, 5 days a week."_

The **best** body part exercise order to *tighten* your buns is:

# LEGS

# SHOULDERS

# BACK

# BICEPS

# TRICEPS

**What? No abs?**

Your ab program will be given to you in Vol. 2 because the focus in this book is reshaping your body as fast as possible and also the 'tummy' work in Vol. 2 is very specialized.

There are many benefits to **flowologee** among them:

Your **POST EXERCISE CONSUMPTION RATE** remains high after your workout **which means** you will be *burning* calories hours <u>**after**</u> your workout.

Your physical **strength** will *increase* because of using resistance. (I recommend resistance bands and body weight for time flexibility.)

Your ***cardiovascular endurance*** will *increase* as I mentioned before because of the blood coursing through your veins after moving through every body part in the "flow."

Your **flexibility** will *increase* because in addition to performing each exercise through a full range of motion, you will be stretching after each session of **30 minutes** and any additional cardio you do...

And most importantly...

you should have **tightened** your *buns, became 'thinner' & **toned*** down by the 30th day!

The first 4 exercises below work on tightening your 'Buns' and legs...
from the peak of your 'Buns', to the area between your 'Buns',
the top of your legs and also tightening up your inner thighs.

## (Legs)
**Hip Raises**
**Hip Raises on Bench**
**Body-weight Squats**
**Wide Body-weight Squats**
**Calf Raises**

## (Shoulders)
**Close Upright Rows**
**Lateral Raises**

## (Back)
**Pullovers**
**Bent Over Rows**

## (Arms)
**Bicep Curls**
**Tricep Kickbacks**

(Go to my website: www.sakanidangeles.com to see videos for each of these exercises.)

# *NOTE*

*Do not rest between exercises. Go from one exercise to another quickly without sacrificing form. One complete run through, from Chest Flyes to Tricep Kickbacks is one complete set.*

## *IMMEDIATELY AFTER YOUR WORKOUT*

### CARDIO:

WHATEVER YOU LIKE FOR 15 MIN MAX
EXAMPLE: RUNNING, SWIMMING, CYCLING, ANYTHING THAT WILL MAKE YOU SWEAT

***NO MORE WEIGHT TRAINING AFTER ABOVE WORKOUT***

### STRETCH:

HOWEVER YOU LIKE... THEN:

*Do this program:*

# 5 DAYS IN A ROW...ONLY!

**9 reps:** legs, shoulders, back, biceps,triceps

## WEEK 1: DO 1 SET FOR 3 DAYS IN A ROW

## WEEK 2: DO 2 SETS FOR 3 DAYS IN A ROW

## WEEK 3: DO 3 SETS FOR 3 DAYS IN A ROW

## WEEK 4: DO 4 SETS FOR 3 DAYS IN A ROW

THE NEXT 3 DAYS ARE **CARDIO ONLY** DAYS. DO WHATEVER CARDIO YOU LIKE FOR THE NEXT 3 DAYS STRAIGHT. **DO NOT** DO THE EXERCISES IN THIS BOOK OR ANY OTHER PROGRAM AS THIS WILL CAUSE YOUR FITNESS LEVEL TO DECREASE.

**SO THIS PROGRAM LOOKS LIKE THIS:**

**3** DAYS 'TIGHT BUNS' WORKOUT
**2** DAYS CARDIO **ONLY**
2 DAYS OFF – NO EXERCISES AT ALL

STOMACH EXERCISES WILL BE COVERED IN VOLUME 2 IN THE SECTION CALLED
'TIGHT TUMMY'.

# **TOOLS:**

You can use small weights. We recommend you use exercise bands.

An *excellent choice* would be the exercise bands which you can purchase at
my website: www.sakanidangeles.com

# What do you eat?

**EAT:** PROTEINS & VEGGIES AFTER THE WORKOUT IN THIS BOOK

## EAT: NO CARBS AFTER 3PM!!!!!

## PROTEINS & VEGGIES ONLY!!!!

(*NO CARBS AFTER 3PM ON THESE 5 DAYS*)

IF STILL HUNGRY ONLY EAT MORE PROTEIN & VEGETABLES

# Additional Guidelines

- Take a picture of yourself on day 1, week 1 **<u>FOR YOURSELF</u>**! You need to see where you are beginning. Also because every artist looks at the raw materials of their masterpieces right? And *you are* a masterpiece in progress!

- Wear sweat or "casual clothes, since the purpose of the training is to force you to sweat and thus make greater demands on your respiratory system for deeper breathing. Breathe through your **NOSE ONLY**. Forget about breathing through your MOUTH during exercise.

- Concentrate on speeding up the routine. Make a focused effort to complete each SET faster than the previous one.

- Your workout should last no more than **<u>30 minutes max.</u>** Time yourself with an alarm clock to go off at 30 minutes passed the time you begin or watch a clock posted nearby. Your cardio workout should be NO more than **<u>15 minutes max.</u>**

- Wait at least **<u>30 minutes before eating.</u>** Eating right after the workout will put greater demands on the digestion system.
- Take a multi-vitamin with breakfast and dinner
- *So exercise, take your shower and then **eat**. Your body will be ready!*

# 'Tight Buns'

## *& fat loss in 30 days or less with flowologee*

## TRAINING LOGS

# 'Tight Buns' in 30 Days...

## Week 1 Training Log

Day:                    Date:                    Time:          Week:

_____            _____              _____  _____

*One set according this program means 1 complete cycle: doing the below exercises one after another until finished with the last exercise on this list.

### Week 1: (1 SET ONLY – 3 DAYS IN A ROW – 2 DAYS CARDIO ONLY – 2 DAYS OFF)

(9 Reps)      **Hip Raises**

(9 Reps      **Hip Raises on Bench**

(9 Reps)      **Body-weight Squats**

(9 Reps)      **Wide Body-weight Squats**

(9 Reps)      **Calf Raises**

(9 Reps)      **Close Upright Rows**

(9 Reps)      **Lat Raises**

(9 Reps)      **Bent Over Rows**

(9 Reps)      **Bicep Curls**

(9 Reps )     **Tricep Kickbacks**

(Go to my website: www.sakanidangeles.com to see videos for each of these exercises.)

**15** Minute Minimum **Cardio** for today:

Exercise: _____Duration: _____

STRETCH: _____ (Good choice: Hurdler's Stretch)

Beginning Time of workout: _____ am/pm

End Time of workout: _____ am/pm

Mood when started workout: _____

Mood when finished with workout: _____

# 'Tight Buns' in 30 Days...

## Week 1 Training Log

**Day:**                 **Date:**                         **Time:**        **Week:**

_____          _____               _____ _____

*One set according this program means 1 complete cycle: doing the below exercises one after another until finished with the last exercise on this list.

### Week 1: (1 SET ONLY – 3 DAYS IN A ROW – 2 DAYS CARDIO ONLY – 2 DAYS OFF)

**(9 Reps)**      **Hip Raises**

**(9 Reps**      **Hip Raises on Bench**

**(9 Reps)**      **Body-weight Squats**

**(9 Reps)**      **Wide Body-weight Squats**

**(9 Reps)**      **Calf Raises**

**(9 Reps)**      **Close Upright Rows**

**(9 Reps)**      **Lat Raises**

**(9 Reps)**      **Bent Over Rows**

**(9 Reps)**      **Bicep Curls**

**(9 Reps )**      **Tricep Kickbacks**

**(Go to my website: www.sakanidangeles.com to see videos for each of these exercises.)**

**15** Minute Minimum **Cardio** for today:

Exercise: _____Duration: _____

STRETCH: _____ (Good choice: Hurdler's Stretch)

Beginning Time of workout: _____ am/pm

End Time of workout: _____ am/pm

Mood when started workout: _____

Mood when finished with workout: _____

# 'Tight Buns' in 30 Days...

## Week 1 Training Log

**Day:**                    **Date:**                    **Time:**        **Week:**

_____        _____        _____ _____

*One set according this program means 1 complete cycle: doing the below exercises one after another until finished with the last exercise on this list.

### Week 1: (1 SET ONLY – 3 DAYS IN A ROW – 2 DAYS CARDIO ONLY – 2 DAYS OFF)

**(9 Reps)**      **Hip Raises**

**(9 Reps**       **Hip Raises on Bench**

**(9 Reps)**      **Body-weight Squats**

**(9 Reps)**      **Wide Body-weight Squats**

**(9 Reps)**      **Calf Raises**

**(9 Reps)**      **Close Upright Rows**

**(9 Reps)**      **Lat Raises**

**(9 Reps)**      **Bent Over Rows**

**(9 Reps)**      **Bicep Curls**

**(9 Reps )**     **Tricep Kickbacks**

(Go to my website: www.sakanidangeles.com to see videos for each of these exercises.)

**15** Minute Minimum **Cardio** for today:

Exercise: _____Duration: _____

STRETCH: _____ (Good choice: Hurdler's Stretch)

Beginning Time of workout: _____ am/pm

End Time of workout: _____ am/pm

Mood when started workout: _____

Mood when finished with workout: _____

# 'Tight Buns' in 30 Days...

## Week 1 Training Log

**Day:** _____  **Date:** _____  **Time:** _____ **Week:** _____

\*One set according this program means 1 complete cycle: doing the below exercises one after another until finished with the last exercise on this list.

### Week 1: (1 SET ONLY – 3 DAYS IN A ROW – 2 DAYS CARDIO ONLY – 2 DAYS OFF)

**(9 Reps)**     **Hip Raises**

**(9 Reps**     **Hip Raises on Bench**

**(9 Reps)**     **Body-weight Squats**

**(9 Reps)**     **Wide Body-weight Squats**

**(9 Reps)**     **Calf Raises**

**(9 Reps)**     **Close Upright Rows**

**(9 Reps)**     **Lat Raises**

**(9 Reps)**     **Bent Over Rows**

**(9 Reps)**     **Bicep Curls**

**(9 Reps )**     **Tricep Kickbacks**

(Go to my website: www.sakanidangeles.com to see videos for each of these exercises.)

**15** Minute Minimum **Cardio** for today:

Exercise: _____Duration: _____

STRETCH: _____ (Good choice: Hurdler's Stretch)

Beginning Time of workout: _____ am/pm

End Time of workout: _____ am/pm

Mood when started workout: _____

Mood when finished with workout: _____

# 'Tight Buns' in 30 Days...

## Week 1 Training Log

Day:                    Date:                    Time:        Week:

_____        _____        _____  _____

*One set according this program means 1 complete cycle: doing the below exercises one after another until finished with the last exercise on this list.

### Week 1: (1 SET ONLY – 3 DAYS IN A ROW – 2 DAYS CARDIO ONLY – 2 DAYS OFF)

(9 Reps)        **Hip Raises**

(9 Reps        **Hip Raises on Bench**

(9 Reps)        **Body-weight Squats**

(9 Reps)        **Wide Body-weight Squats**

(9 Reps)        **Calf Raises**

(9 Reps)        **Close Upright Rows**

(9 Reps)        **Lat Raises**

(9 Reps)        **Bent Over Rows**

(9 Reps)        **Bicep Curls**

(9 Reps )        **Tricep Kickbacks**

(Go to my website: www.sakanidangeles.com to see videos for each of these exercises.)

**15** Minute Minimum **Cardio** for today:

Exercise: _____Duration: _____

STRETCH: _____ (Good choice: Hurdler's Stretch)

Beginning Time of workout: _____ am/pm

End Time of workout: _____ am/pm

Mood when started workout: _____

Mood when finished with workout: _____

# 'Tight Buns' in 30 Days...

## Week 2 Training Log

**Day:**              **Date:**              **Time:**        **Week:**

_____          _____          _____ _____

*One set according this program means 1 complete cycle: doing the below exercises one after another until finished with the last exercise on this list.

### Week 2: (2 SETS ONLY– 3 DAYS IN A ROW – 2 DAYS CARDIO ONLY – 2 DAYS OFF)

**(9 Reps)**      **Hip Raises**

**(9 Reps**      **Hip Raises on Bench**

**(9 Reps)**      **Body-weight Squats**

**(9 Reps)**      **Wide Body-weight Squats**

**(9 Reps)**      **Calf Raises**

**(9 Reps)**      **Close Upright Rows**

**(9 Reps)**      **Lat Raises**

**(9 Reps)**      **Bent Over Rows**

**(9 Reps)**      **Bicep Curls**

**(9 Reps )**      **Tricep Kickbacks**

**(Go to my website: www.sakanidangeles.com to see videos for each of these exercises.)**

**15** Minute Minimum **Cardio** for today:

Exercise: _____Duration: _____

STRETCH: _____ (Good choice: Hurdler's Stretch)

Beginning Time of workout: _____ am/pm

End Time of workout: _____ am/pm

Mood when started workout: _____

Mood when finished with workout: _____

# 'Tight Buns' in 30 Days...

## Week 2 Training Log

**Day:**                    **Date:**                    **Time:**        **Week:**

_____          _____          _____  _____

*One set according this program means 1 complete cycle: doing the below exercises one after another until finished with the last exercise on this list.

### Week 2: (2 SETS ONLY– 3 DAYS IN A ROW – 2 DAYS CARDIO ONLY – 2 DAYS OFF)

(9 Reps)    **Hip Raises**

(9 Reps    **Hip Raises on Bench**

(9 Reps)    **Body-weight Squats**

(9 Reps)    **Wide Body-weight Squats**

(9 Reps)    **Calf Raises**

(9 Reps)    **Close Upright Rows**

(9 Reps)    **Lat Raises**

(9 Reps)    **Bent Over Rows**

(9 Reps)    **Bicep Curls**

(9 Reps )    **Tricep Kickbacks**

(Go to my website: www.sakanidangeles.com to see videos for each of these exercises.)

**15** Minute Minimum **Cardio** for today:

Exercise: _____Duration: _____

STRETCH: _____ (Good choice: Hurdler's Stretch)

Beginning Time of workout: _____ am/pm

End Time of workout: _____ am/pm

Mood when started workout: _____

Mood when finished with workout: _____

# 'Tight Buns' in 30 Days...

## Week 2 Training Log

**Day:**             **Date:**                   **Time:**         **Week:**

_____         _____         _____ _____

*One set according this program means 1 complete cycle: doing the below exercises one after another until finished with the last exercise on this list.

### Week 2: (2 SETS ONLY– 3 DAYS IN A ROW – 2 DAYS CARDIO ONLY – 2 DAYS OFF)

**(9 Reps)**      **Hip Raises**

**(9 Reps**      **Hip Raises on Bench**

**(9 Reps)**      **Body-weight Squats**

**(9 Reps)**      **Wide Body-weight Squats**

**(9 Reps)**      **Calf Raises**

**(9 Reps)**      **Close Upright Rows**

**(9 Reps)**      **Lat Raises**

**(9 Reps)**      **Bent Over Rows**

**(9 Reps)**      **Bicep Curls**

**(9 Reps )**      **Tricep Kickbacks**

(Go to my website: www.sakanidangeles.com to see videos for each of these exercises.)

**15** Minute Minimum **Cardio** for today:

Exercise: _____Duration: _____

STRETCH: _____ (Good choice: Hurdler's Stretch)

Beginning Time of workout: _____ am/pm

End Time of workout: _____ am/pm

Mood when started workout: _____

Mood when finished with workout: _____

# 'Tight Buns' in 30 Days...

## Week 2 Training Log

**Day:** _____ **Date:** _____ **Time:** _____ **Week:** _____

*One set according this program means 1 complete cycle: doing the below exercises one after another until finished with the last exercise on this list.

### Week 2: (2 SETS ONLY– 3 DAYS IN A ROW – 2 DAYS CARDIO ONLY – 2 DAYS OFF)

(9 Reps)   **Hip Raises**

(9 Reps   **Hip Raises on Bench**

(9 Reps)   **Body-weight Squats**

(9 Reps)   **Wide Body-weight Squats**

(9 Reps)   **Calf Raises**

(9 Reps)   **Close Upright Rows**

(9 Reps)   **Lat Raises**

(9 Reps)   **Bent Over Rows**

(9 Reps)   **Bicep Curls**

(9 Reps )   **Tricep Kickbacks**

(Go to my website: www.sakanidangeles.com to see videos for each of these exercises.)

**15** Minute Minimum **Cardio** for today:

Exercise: _____Duration: _____

STRETCH: _____ (Good choice: Hurdler's Stretch)

Beginning Time of workout: _____ am/pm

End Time of workout: _____ am/pm

Mood when started workout: _____

Mood when finished with workout: _____

# 'Tight Buns' in 30 Days...

## Week 2 Training Log

**Day:**             **Date:**                **Time:**        **Week:**

_____            _____           _____ _____

*One set according this program means 1 complete cycle: doing the below exercises one after another until finished with the last exercise on this list.

### Week 2: (2 SETS ONLY– 3 DAYS IN A ROW – 2 DAYS CARDIO ONLY – 2 DAYS OFF)

**(9 Reps)**      **Hip Raises**

**(9 Reps**      **Hip Raises on Bench**

**(9 Reps)**      **Body-weight Squats**

**(9 Reps)**      **Wide Body-weight Squats**

**(9 Reps)**      **Calf Raises**

**(9 Reps)**      **Close Upright Rows**

**(9 Reps)**      **Lat Raises**

**(9 Reps)**      **Bent Over Rows**

**(9 Reps)**      **Bicep Curls**

**(9 Reps )**      **Tricep Kickbacks**

**(Go to my website: www.sakanidangeles.com to see videos for each of these exercises.)**

**15** Minute Minimum **Cardio** for today:

Exercise: _____Duration: _____

STRETCH: _____ (Good choice: Hurdler's Stretch)

Beginning Time of workout: _____ am/pm

End Time of workout: _____ am/pm

Mood when started workout: _____

Mood when finished with workout: _____

# 'Tight Buns' in 30 Days...

## Week 3 Training Log

**Day:** _____ **Date:** _____ **Time:** _____ **Week:** _____

*One set according this program means 1 complete cycle: doing the below exercises one after another until finished with the last exercise on this list.

### Week 3: (3 SETS ONLY– 3 DAYS IN A ROW – 2 DAYS CARDIO ONLY – 2 DAYS OFF)

(9 Reps)    **Hip Raises**

(9 Reps    **Hip Raises on Bench**

(9 Reps)    **Body-weight Squats**

(9 Reps)    **Wide Body-weight Squats**

(9 Reps)    **Calf Raises**

(9 Reps)    **Close Upright Rows**

(9 Reps)    **Lat Raises**

(9 Reps)    **Bent Over Rows**

(9 Reps)    **Bicep Curls**

(9 Reps )    **Tricep Kickbacks**

(Go to my website: www.sakanidangeles.com to see videos for each of these exercises.)

**15** Minute Minimum **Cardio** for today:

Exercise: _____Duration: _____

STRETCH: _____ (Good choice: Hurdler's Stretch)

Beginning Time of workout: _____ am/pm

End Time of workout: _____ am/pm

Mood when started workout: _____

Mood when finished with workout: _____

# 'Tight Buns' in 30 Days...

## Week 3 Training Log

**Day:** _____ **Date:** _____ **Time:** _____ **Week:** _____

*One set according this program means 1 complete cycle: doing the below exercises one after another until finished with the last exercise on this list.

### Week 3: (3 SETS ONLY– 3 DAYS IN A ROW – 2 DAYS CARDIO ONLY – 2 DAYS OFF)

**(9 Reps)**    **Hip Raises**

**(9 Reps**    **Hip Raises on Bench**

**(9 Reps)**    **Body-weight Squats**

**(9 Reps)**    **Wide Body-weight Squats**

**(9 Reps)**    **Calf Raises**

**(9 Reps)**    **Close Upright Rows**

**(9 Reps)**    **Lat Raises**

**(9 Reps)**    **Bent Over Rows**

**(9 Reps)**    **Bicep Curls**

**(9 Reps )**    **Tricep Kickbacks**

(Go to my website: www.sakanidangeles.com to see videos for each of these exercises.)

**15** Minute Minimum **Cardio** for today:

Exercise: _____Duration: _____

STRETCH: _____ (Good choice: Hurdler's Stretch)

Beginning Time of workout: _____ am/pm

End Time of workout: _____ am/pm

Mood when started workout: _____

Mood when finished with workout: _____

# 'Tight Buns' in 30 Days...

## Week 3 Training Log

Day:                    Date:                    Time:        Week:

_____            _____            _____  _____

*One set according this program means 1 complete cycle: doing the below exercises one after another until finished with the last exercise on this list.

### Week 3: (3 SETS ONLY– 3 DAYS IN A ROW – 2 DAYS CARDIO ONLY – 2 DAYS OFF)

(9 Reps)       **Hip Raises**

(9 Reps        **Hip Raises on Bench**

(9 Reps)       **Body-weight Squats**

(9 Reps)       **Wide Body-weight Squats**

(9 Reps)       **Calf Raises**

(9 Reps)       **Close Upright Rows**

(9 Reps)       **Lat Raises**

(9 Reps)       **Bent Over Rows**

(9 Reps)       **Bicep Curls**

(9 Reps )      **Tricep Kickbacks**

(Go to my website: www.sakanidangeles.com to see videos for each of these exercises.)

**15** Minute Minimum **Cardio** for today:

Exercise: _____Duration: _____

STRETCH: _____ (Good choice: Hurdler's Stretch)

Beginning Time of workout: _____ am/pm

End Time of workout: _____ am/pm

Mood when started workout: _____

Mood when finished with workout: _____

# 'Tight Buns' in 30 Days...

## Week 3 Training Log

**Day:**                   **Date:**                 **Time:**      **Week:**

_____         _____         _____ _____

*One set according this program means 1 complete cycle: doing the below exercises one after another until finished with the last exercise on this list.

### Week 3: (3 SETS ONLY– 3 DAYS IN A ROW – 2 DAYS CARDIO ONLY – 2 DAYS OFF)

**(9 Reps)**       **Hip Raises**

**(9 Reps**        **Hip Raises on Bench**

**(9 Reps)**       **Body-weight Squats**

**(9 Reps)**       **Wide Body-weight Squats**

**(9 Reps)**       **Calf Raises**

**(9 Reps)**       **Close Upright Rows**

**(9 Reps)**       **Lat Raises**

**(9 Reps)**       **Bent Over Rows**

**(9 Reps)**       **Bicep Curls**

**(9 Reps )**      **Tricep Kickbacks**

**(Go to my website: www.sakanidangeles.com to see videos for each of these exercises.)**

**15** Minute Minimum **Cardio** for today:

Exercise: _____Duration: _____

STRETCH: _____ (Good choice: Hurdler's Stretch)

Beginning Time of workout: _____ am/pm

End Time of workout: _____ am/pm

Mood when started workout: _____

Mood when finished with workout: _____

# 'Tight Buns' in 30 Days...

## Week 3 Training Log

**Day:**                    **Date:**                         **Time:**        **Week:**

_____        _____          _____ _____

*One set according this program means 1 complete cycle: doing the below exercises one after another until finished with the last exercise on this list.

### Week 3: (3 SETS ONLY– 3 DAYS IN A ROW – 2 DAYS CARDIO ONLY – 2 DAYS OFF)

(9 Reps)        **Hip Raises**

(9 Reps        **Hip Raises on Bench**

(9 Reps)        **Body-weight Squats**

(9 Reps)        **Wide Body-weight Squats**

(9 Reps)        **Calf Raises**

(9 Reps)        **Close Upright Rows**

(9 Reps)        **Lat Raises**

(9 Reps)        **Bent Over Rows**

(9 Reps)        **Bicep Curls**

(9 Reps )       **Tricep Kickbacks**

(Go to my website: www.sakanidangeles.com to see videos for each of these exercises.)

**15** Minute Minimum **Cardio** for today:

Exercise: _____Duration: _____

STRETCH: _____ (Good choice: Hurdler's Stretch)

Beginning Time of workout: _____ am/pm

End Time of workout: _____ am/pm

Mood when started workout: _____

Mood when finished with workout: _____

# 'Tight Buns' in 30 Days...

## Week 4 Training Log

Day:                    Date:                    Time:        Week:

_____        _____        _____  _____

*One set according this program means 1 complete cycle: doing the below exercises one after another until finished with the last exercise on this list.

### Week 4: (4 SETS ONLY– 3 DAYS IN A ROW – 2 DAYS CARDIO ONLY – 2 DAYS OFF)

(9 Reps)      Hip Raises

(9 Reps       Hip Raises on Bench

(9 Reps)      Body-weight Squats

(9 Reps)      Wide Body-weight Squats

(9 Reps)      Calf Raises

(9 Reps)      Close Upright Rows

(9 Reps)      Lat Raises

(9 Reps)      Bent Over Rows

(9 Reps)      Bicep Curls

(9 Reps )     Tricep Kickbacks

(Go to my website: www.sakanidangeles.com to see videos for each of these exercises.)

**15** Minute Minimum **Cardio** for today:

Exercise: _____Duration: _____

STRETCH: _____ (Good choice: Hurdler's Stretch)

Beginning Time of workout: _____ am/pm

End Time of workout: _____ am/pm

Mood when started workout: _____

Mood when finished with workout: _____

# 'Tight Buns' in 30 Days...

## Week 4 Training Log

**Day:**            **Date:**            **Time:**      **Week:**

_____            _____            _____ _____

\*One set according this program means 1 complete cycle: doing the below exercises one after another until finished with the last exercise on this list.

**Week 4: (4 SETS ONLY– 3 DAYS IN A ROW – 2 DAYS CARDIO ONLY – 2 DAYS OFF)**

**(9 Reps)**      **Hip Raises**

**(9 Reps**      **Hip Raises on Bench**

**(9 Reps)**      **Body-weight Squats**

**(9 Reps)**      **Wide Body-weight Squats**

**(9 Reps)**      **Calf Raises**

**(9 Reps)**      **Close Upright Rows**

**(9 Reps)**      **Lat Raises**

**(9 Reps)**      **Bent Over Rows**

**(9 Reps)**      **Bicep Curls**

**(9 Reps )**      **Tricep Kickbacks**

(Go to my website: www.sakanidangeles.com to see videos for each of these exercises.)

**15** Minute Minimum **Cardio** for today:

Exercise: _____Duration: _____

STRETCH: _____ (Good choice: Hurdler's Stretch)

Beginning Time of workout: _____ am/pm

End Time of workout: _____ am/pm

Mood when started workout: _____

Mood when finished with workout: _____

# 'Tight Buns' in 30 Days...

## Week 4 Training Log

**Day:** _____  **Date:** _____  **Time:** _____  **Week:** _____

*One set according this program means 1 complete cycle: doing the below exercises one after another until finished with the last exercise on this list.

### Week 4: (4 SETS ONLY– 3 DAYS IN A ROW – 2 DAYS CARDIO ONLY – 2 DAYS OFF)

**(9 Reps)**     **Hip Raises**

**(9 Reps**      **Hip Raises on Bench**

**(9 Reps)**     **Body-weight Squats**

**(9 Reps)**     **Wide Body-weight Squats**

**(9 Reps)**     **Calf Raises**

**(9 Reps)**     **Close Upright Rows**

**(9 Reps)**     **Lat Raises**

**(9 Reps)**     **Bent Over Rows**

**(9 Reps)**     **Bicep Curls**

**(9 Reps )**    **Tricep Kickbacks**

**(Go to my website: www.sakanidangeles.com to see videos for each of these exercises.)**

**15** Minute Minimum **Cardio** for today:

Exercise: _____Duration: _____

STRETCH: _____ (Good choice: Hurdler's Stretch)

Beginning Time of workout: _____ am/pm

End Time of workout: _____ am/pm

Mood when started workout: _____

Mood when finished with workout: _____

# 'Tight Buns' in 30 Days...

## Week 4 Training Log

**Day:** _____ **Date:** _____ **Time:** _____ **Week:** _____

*One set according this program means 1 complete cycle: doing the below exercises one after another until finished with the last exercise on this list.

### Week 4: (4 SETS ONLY– 3 DAYS IN A ROW – 2 DAYS CARDIO ONLY – 2 DAYS OFF)

**(9 Reps)**    **Hip Raises**

**(9 Reps**    **Hip Raises on Bench**

**(9 Reps)**    **Body-weight Squats**

**(9 Reps)**    **Wide Body-weight Squats**

**(9 Reps)**    **Calf Raises**

**(9 Reps)**    **Close Upright Rows**

**(9 Reps)**    **Lat Raises**

**(9 Reps)**    **Bent Over Rows**

**(9 Reps)**    **Bicep Curls**

**(9 Reps )**    **Tricep Kickbacks**

(Go to my website: www.sakanidangeles.com to see videos for each of these exercises.)

**15** Minute Minimum **Cardio** for today:

Exercise: _____Duration: _____

STRETCH: _____ (Good choice: Hurdler's Stretch)

Beginning Time of workout: _____ am/pm

End Time of workout: _____ am/pm

Mood when started workout: _____

Mood when finished with workout: _____

# 'Tight Buns' in 30 Days...

## Week 4 Training Log

**Day:**          **Date:**                    **Time:**        **Week:**

_____          _____                    _____   _____

*One set according this program means 1 complete cycle: doing the below exercises one after another until finished with the last exercise on this list.

### Week 4: (4 SETS ONLY– 3 DAYS IN A ROW – 2 DAYS CARDIO ONLY – 2 DAYS OFF)

(9 Reps)     **Hip Raises**

(9 Reps     **Hip Raises on Bench**

(9 Reps)     **Body-weight Squats**

(9 Reps)     **Wide Body-weight Squats**

(9 Reps)     **Calf Raises**

(9 Reps)     **Close Upright Rows**

(9 Reps)     **Lat Raises**

(9 Reps)     **Bent Over Rows**

(9 Reps)     **Bicep Curls**

(9 Reps )    **Tricep Kickbacks**

(Go to my website: www.sakanidangeles.com to see videos for each of these exercises.)

**15** Minute Minimum **Cardio** for today:

Exercise: _____Duration: _____

STRETCH: _____ (Good choice: Hurdler's Stretch)

Beginning Time of workout: _____ am/pm

End Time of workout: _____ am/pm

Mood when started workout: _____

Mood when finished with workout: _____

*"Action without thinking is the cause of every failure."*
*Peter Drucker*

# Sakani D'Angeles

# Acknowledgments...

First, I must thank **God** for the inspiration to teach this information that has keep and continues to keep me healthy and looking younger every day.

*Thank you for having Mercy on me.*

**Dad & Mom**
Always encouraging, top shelf, amazing parents who I am happy to have.
**Ali Hakeem**
Thanks for the support and being my little brother. Team work makes the dream work.
E.A., Mi ese y papa de mi corazones... Gracias por todo,
**Ernesto Ancira, Jr.**
It was an honor to spend the little time I have and look to my encounter with you as the fuel and fire for pushing forward.
**Yi-Chun Tricia Lin**
Your inspiration and encouragement for me to write was a seed that I am glad you planted. I am honored to still have you in my life.

**Everyone who I have met. Period. I am inspired by all.**

# Sakani D'Angeles

# 'Tight Buns'

## *& fat loss in 30 days or less with flowologee*

Special books or book excerpts can be created to fit specific needs.
For more information & details Visit my website at: WWW.sakanidangeles.com

This book contains the complete text of the hardcover edition.
If you find any errors please email me at sakaniflowcoach@gmail.com

# Who am I?

And why...

The reason for this small book is to make simple for you what many in our industry make complicated.

A member of the Morgan family was heard saying, (paraphrased), "You will never be successful if you make the complicated simple. You must make the simple complicated." It is sad that this is the American way. People know that simple is better but because we are overwhelmed with complex is better we refuse the truth and the truth is always simple.

While going to college in New York City I began training in Wing Chun Kung Fu, the first style of martial arts studied by the late Bruce Lee, with my cousin and uncle and so began my fascination with Bruce Lee. I have always been thin with an "ectomorph" body type. Long legs, long arms, small waist and high metabolism. I could not identify with the big muscled types.... I could identify with Bruce Lee... The gracefulness... the elegance... the quickness... the stamina... the pleasing side effect of the beauty of his body. To look good and to do good... I wanted that. This was the beginning of the quest.

At the time there was not much information on how he trained his body so I began using my body as the laboratory. Trying to make myself better became my passion and then... because I love sharing and teaching, sharing and teaching this to others so that they can be better humans, fathers, mothers, people... became my other passion. I have become excellent at quickly enhancing the human body. I am living proof. And then there was Regina...

She was my first living proof that what I had compiled, based on scientific information only, was a quick way of shaping, toning, losing fat and enhancing the human body. Her family thought she was on crack! That she was on drugs because of how fast she toned down and how much more energy she had! I thought... wow... I have something here... And now you have it!

# 'Tight Buns'

*& fat loss in 30 days or less with flowologee*

©

## DBC PUBLISHING GLOBAL

www.sakanidangeles.com

www.ingramcontent.com/pod-product-compliance
Lightning Source LLC
Chambersburg PA
CBHW080613290526
45790CB00007B/2756